Exercises
for
Airplanes

(and Other Confined Spaces)

Exercises
for
Airplanes
(and Other Confined Spaces)

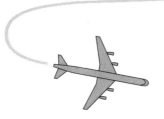

Janet Diamond

Excalibur Publishing
New York

Published by:
Excalibur Publishing Inc.
511 Avenue of the Americas, Suite 392
New York, New York 10011

Cover and graphic design: Kara Glasgold, Griffin Design
Illustrations: Zipora Schulz

The ideas and suggestions contained in this book are not intended
to replace the services of a trained health professional. If you have
any serious or long-term problems or are currently undergoing any
course of medical treatment, consult your health professional before
trying any of the suggestions in this book. Any use of the exercises
and treatments in this book are at the reader's discretion, and neither
the author nor publisher can be held responsible for any adverse
reactions to any exercises or remedies contained herein.

Library of Congress Cataloging in Publication Data

Diamond, Janet.
  Exercises for airplanes (and other confined spaces) / Janet
Diamond.
      p.   cm.
  Includes bibliographical references.
  ISBN 1-885064-03-9 (pbk.)
    1. Isometric exercise. 2. Air travel--Health aspects.
3. Stretching exercises. 4. Travel--Health aspects. I. Title.
RA781.2.D52 1996
613.7'149--dc20   96-27726
                                                              CIP

Printed in the United States of America

10 9 8 7 6 5 4 3 2 1

To Michael Roach, the frequent flier Geshe

Contents

Acknowledgments

The author wishes to thank her parents, Frank and Paulette, for their bottomless generosity, Paul Wesley for his support and enthusiasm, and Sharon Good for conceiving this project and guiding it along the way.

Introduction

In December 1994, while engaged in a book promotion tour, former vice president Dan Quayle suffered a pulmonary embolism, or blood clot in the lungs, a condition which cuts off blood supply to the lungs and can be fatal if untreated. He was hospitalized for over a week, and his doctors believed that the first clot originated in his right leg, due to prolonged sitting on airplanes.

When people sit in a cross-legged position for long periods, the circulation from the veins of the leg towards the heart slows down, and clotting may ensue. Upon his release from the hospital, the former vice president advised others to get up and walk around the aisles at regular intervals.

I discussed this event with Sharon Good, an editor at Excalibur Publishing, who mentioned that she had wanted to collaborate with a physical therapist on a book about exercises people could do on airplanes and in other confined spaces. At the time, I had been employed for several years as a massage therapist at several first class hotels in New York. Many of my clients were stressed-out business travelers who had spent long hours on planes, carrying luggage, and experiencing jet lag, sore muscles, and general fatigue. Because of my background in massage therapy and dance, as well as writing, I offered to work on the project. That's how this book was born.

While Mr. Quayle had a specific medical condition that most of us may never face, anyone who has ever sat on a plane for more than a few hours can testify to feeling sore, achy, uncomfortable, or just pain stir crazy from all those hours of sitting in a confined space. This book is dedicated to those travelers everywhere. May it provide relief!

How To Use This Book

This book was created to provide physical exercises, self-massage techniques, and dietary and supplemental aids to relieve the discomforts of air travel. It provides a general guideline for travelers to exercise on airplanes and in other confined spaces, such as train or bus seats, or even to take a break at your computer workstation.

We begin with a general warm-up sequence, including gentle stretches for the body as a whole. Then we focus on specific areas of the body to stretch and strengthen. Select exercises that appeal to you and address your particular needs, or refer to the suggested routines on pages 31-32 .

Within each body part, the exercises require varying levels of strength, flexibility, and coordination. Be aware that needs and physical capabilities may vary widely according to the individual. As with any exercise regimen, be sensitive to your body's response to these suggestions, and do them with discretion. If something is hurting, stop the exercise or do it more gently. Never force anything. If you have injuries or disabilities, consult with your doctor or other health professional before implementing these exercises.

There is a special section devoted to visualizations for relaxation and to improve posture. If, however, at any point you find wish to do any of the exercises, but feel uncomfortable performing them in a public place, you can still reap benefit from visualizing that you are executing them. This technique has been done successfully with athletes to prepare them for competition. However, many of these exercises are very contained and can easily be performed in your seat without anyone else being aware of what you are doing, and once you have learned them, you will be able to perform many of them effortlessly while engaged in other activities such as watching the movie or reading. But even the exercises that are more conspicuous will probably get few stares, as our culture has become very fitness-oriented.

And finally, suggestions are offered to help you cope with the side effects of travel, including jet lag, dehydration, motion sickness, upset stomach, diarrhea, constipation, insomnia, alertness and energy, sinus problems, and fear of flying. Foods and over-the-counter remedies are mentioned, along with several alternative therapies, such as herbs and homeopathy. Again, numerous suggestions are made so that you can choose the method that appeals to you and the particular remedy that works best.

General Warm-Up

#1 — Sitting Up Straight

Unfortunately, train and plane seats are poorly designed in terms of body mechanics. They tend to encourage you to either slump, which causes your chest to cave in and your lower back to compress, or to arch your back, which puts strain on your lower back. Neither is desirable. To compensate for this imbalance, it is best to lean slightly forward, hold the stomach in without straining, and lift the bottom of your rib cage up and out of your spine.

Try to sit erect. Feel your spine getting longer. A good way to feel this is to imagine your spine as a piece of elastic thread being pulled out from the top of your head at the same time that it is being pulled at its base. You should not hold your body in a way that feels rigid or static, but rather feel like you are growing. If a pillow or other soft object is available, you may find it helpful to place it behind your lower back for added support. (I sometimes use a day pack for this purpose.) Take a deep breath and let it out.

#2 — Wake-up

After sitting awhile, you'll feel rather sluggish. This exercise will help wake up your body. With a loose fist, gently tap your muscles. You can start with your neck and shoulders, then work your way down the top of your arm, around your wrist, and up the inside. Lift your arm and tap down the side of your body, across your waist and up the center of the chest, tapping a little more at the shoulder if you wish. Repeat on the other side. Tap your lower back and butt. Tap your legs, going down the outside and up the inside, or down the front and up the back (if you can maneuver it!). You can also gently tap your face and head with your fingertips. This is a good one to start with!

#3 — Spinal Twist

Staying erect, place your left hand on the outside of your right leg just below the knee, and twist your spine to the right. You can also use the armrest to get better leverage. You may hear some cracking. This is no cause to worry, and many associate this sound with a release. Repeat on the other side.

#4 — Leg and Hip Stretch

Keeping the left foot firmly planted on the floor, lift the entire right foot off the floor. Let your knee come up as high as possible, without banging into anything. Pull your knee toward your chest and hold briefly. Repeat on the other side. This will help limber up your hip sockets.

#5 — Waist Lengthener

Grab the right armrest with your right arm. Now stretch the left hand towards the floor. Let your weight lean into this position. Repeat on the other side.

#6 — Arm Stretches

Lift your arms as high over your head as possible without hitting anything. Bend your elbows if necessary. Stretch first the right arm, and then the left, as though reaching for something over your head. If you're lucky enough to get an aisle seat, you should be able to do this one without any restrictions.

#7 — Breathing

✈ This exercise promotes healing and is taken from Tibetan medicine. Visualize someone you admire greatly. See them holding a lapis lazuli stone (it is a deep blue) or other crystal or precious metal that you find beautiful. Or if you prefer, simply see the color you are drawn to. Take a deep breath and see the beautiful, vibrant color going into you, filling you with energy, confidence, and joy. When you exhale, see gray clouds of smoke leaving your body, taking with it any emotional or physical discomfort or negativity. Repeat two or more times.

✈ A variation on this is to visualize breathing in each of the seven colors of the rainbow (red, orange, yellow, green, blue, indigo, and violet) and seeing that color light filling your body.

✈ Here is another exercise you can do to calm down when you are feeling stress. It is taken from Vipassana and Zen meditation methods. Breathe normally, but as you inhale, count to yourself the number #1. As you exhale, count to yourself the number #2. Repeat starting at #1 again. If you feel your mind wandering, do not get upset; just calmly bring yourself back to number #1. Try to do this for five minutes. This technique is helpful when you are feeling agitated.

Exercises by Body Parts

Now we will group exercises for various body parts. Feel free to skip around. You may prefer to work from the top down, from the bottom up, in random order, or focus on a particular area of the body. Do some or all of these exercises in any order that feels good to you.

~ Shoulders ~

From other sections — #2, #6, #10, #18.

#8 — Shoulder Lifts and Drops

Lift your shoulders towards your ears, bring them up tightly, and then drop them. When you drop them, do just that, let them really drop, rather than pushing them down by exerting a lot of control. Exhale when you do it, and let go of any residual tension. Repeat three times. Now lift and drop just the right shoulder four times. Repeat on the left.

#9 — Shoulder Rolls

Staying erect, move your shoulders in a circular motion. Start toward the front and work your way in a smooth circular motion, continuing up, and then finally back and down. Reverse this motion starting back first, then up, and finally forward and down. Do four traveling back, and then four traveling forward. Then do one shoulder at a time — four rotations on the right traveling back, then four on the left. Then repeat traveling backward — four on the right, then four on the left. Take a deep breath and really let it out.

#10 — Neck and Shoulder Release

Sitting upright, release your arms and hands so that they hang straight and loosely by your sides. While pressing your shoulders down, rotate your right arm out, so that your thumb points back behind you. Your right elbow should be facing in toward your body. Press outward with the muscles under your right armpit. To check if they are engaged correctly, you can place your left hand under your armpit. Tense and then release the muscles under the armpit. Repeat two more times. Try it on the other side. After doing this, you should feel a release in your upper body. Note that this is very subtle and may take time to perfect, because it involves isolating certain muscles, and you should not strain to do this.

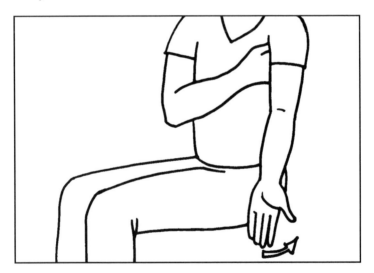

What this does — Most of us tend to hold tension in our neck and shoulders. This exercise redirects the tension to the long skeletal muscles that support our back (latissimus dorsi). This allows us to release the tension in the neck and shoulders and improve our skeletal alignment.

~ BACK ~

From other sections — #1, #3, #5, #37.
You may want to do these exercises again to help realign the spine and lengthen the back.

#11 — Back Release

This exercise will work for those who are small enough or have a bulkhead seat. Make sure your tray table is securely fastened before you try this one! Sitting straight, with your feet flat on the floor, bend forward at the waist, letting your chest drop onto the front of your thighs. (If you don't have enough room to bend completely forward, try curling your back as far forward as you can without hitting your head. You'll still get some benefit.) Let your head drop forward and your hands drop to the floor. Gently shake the shoulders and then the neck in this position. Try moving your head first forward and backward, and then from right to left. Be very passive, and let gravity do the work. When you're ready to come up, curl up from the base of the spine, unraveling one vertebrae at a time, until you are upright. This is an excellent stretch for the neck and back.

#12 — Pelvic Tilts

Sitting upright, with both feet flat on the floor, hold your stomach in, slightly tighten the buttocks, and push your sit bones forward. You should not slide forward in your seat if you are doing this correctly. This is a subtle move, but will greatly reduce lower back pain if done correctly and on a regular basis.

#13 — Leg Isometrics

Sitting erect, bring the insides of your legs tightly together, so that your thighs, lower legs, and ankles, are touching each other. Hold your stomach in firmly, while clenching your buttocks, and press your thighs together tightly. Hold for thirty seconds and release. Then try to hold for longer periods. This works the abdomen, buttocks, and inner thigh muscles, improves posture, and takes pressure off the lower back.

#14 — Rib Cage Isolations

Press your rib cage forward. Bring it back to center. Pull it in so that it goes behind you, and back to center. Repeat two times. Now push it to the right, then to center, and to the left, and center. Repeat two more times. Next, slowly move it in a continuous smooth circle, starting at the right, continuing forward, left, back, and right. Reverse this motion, starting left, moving forward, right, back, and left. Do three circles in each direction. This releases tension and gives you freedom of movement in the upper body.

~ HANDS AND ARMS ~

From other sections — #2, #5, #6, #10.

#15 — Hand Strengthener

Make a fist with each hand. Squeeze hard and hold for a count of five. Then stretch your fingers as wide and as long as possible. Hold for a count of five. Repeat. Shake your hands out from side to side, and from back to front.

#16 — Hand Grip and Pectoral Strengthener

✈ Grab each armrest. Place each thumb on the inside surface and the remaining fingers on the outside. Squeeze the handle with your whole hand. Release. Squeeze and release. Repeat two more times. Shake your hands out.

✈ Place your forearms inside the armrests. Press your elbows out and against the inside surface of the arm rest. Release. Repeat three times. This strengthens your pectoral (chest) muscles.

✈ Move your arms slightly forward, so that your forearms cross in front of you. Again press your elbows out and against the inner surface of the armrests. Repeat this three times. You should feel your arm extensors (the muscles on the outer surface of your arms, including the triceps) working.

✈ Place your elbows on the armrests. Join the palms of your hands together in the position used for prayer. This position might come in handy on rocky flights! Press your palms tightly together and release. Repeat several times. This strengthens the flexor muscles of your upper arms (those on the inner surface, including the biceps), as well as the pectoral (chest) muscles.

#17 — Wrist and Hand Release

This is actually a series of stretches.

✈ Shake your wrists out, moving them from side to side. Now shake them out, moving them from front to back.

✈ Rotate them so that both wrists circle, first in an outward, then an inward direction.

✈ Starting with the fingers straight out, curl the fingers in, one by one starting with the pinky and ending with the thumb, until your hand is in a loose fist, then stretch them out again finger by finger, again starting with the pinky and ending with the thumb. The wrists will twist slightly. Repeat several times.

✦ Circle each finger first in a clockwise direction, then reverse.

✦ Bring the pinky of each hand to touch the thumb of the same hand. Then stretch them back away from each other. Release and repeat. In a similar fashion, join each of the other fingers to the thumb of the same hand, and then stretch away.

✦ Place your left palm face up and keep your fingers straight. Place all the fingers of the right hand, except the thumb, across the fingers of the left hand at a right angle to them. Let the thumb of your right hand rest underneath the left hand. Using your right hand, gently press the fingers of your left hand back, so that your palm stretches (see diagram). Repeat on the other side. Shake out your hands.

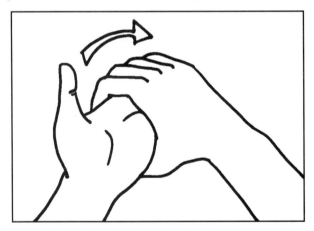

✦ With your tray table open, "let your fingers do the walking." Start them at the edge of the tray closest to you and walk them forward to the other end of the tray. Then walk them back.

#18 — Neck, Shoulder, and Arm Self-Massage

Using your right hand, you'll massage your left side. Begin by massaging the muscles in your neck, starting at the hairline. Slowly work your way down your shoulder, upper arm, elbow, and forearm, down to the wrist. Spend a little more time on spots that may feel sore or tense. Repeat on the other side. To complete, follow this up with exercise #19. You'll feel much lighter and more relaxed after this one!

#19 — Hand Self-Massage and Reflexology

Reflexology is a healing art based on the idea that there are reflex points on the feet that relate to the organs, glands, and body parts. At the turn of the century, Dr. William Fitzgerald developed zone theory, which proposed that different body parts relate to one another, and that by applying pressure to one area, another area could be anesthetized. In the 1930's, Eunice Ingham, a physiotherapist and believer in the theory, discovered that of all the body parts, the feet were the most responsive. She mapped out the entire body on the feet and discovered that by stimulating specific points on the soles of the feet and the palms of the hands, one can rectify imbalances in the whole body, thereby relieving stress and improving well-being. While it is helpful to learn this healing art and study charts, it is possible to treat oneself without knowing specific points, just by being sensitive to one's own body.

✈ Apply some lotion to your hands. Often the air on planes is very dry, so the moisture will do you good. Gently rub it in, covering the whole palm surface and the fingers. Rub the skin between the base of the fingers; according to Tibetan medicine, this will release toxins and help to energize you. It is especially helpful to rub the spot on the back of the hand between the thumb and index finger. According to shiatsu, this area pertains to the large intestine meridian (or energy pathway), which will help with digestion, headaches, and sinus problems. The corresponding spot on the palm surface pertains to the lung meridian. These two points can be rubbed simultaneously by placing the thumb and index fingers of one hand on these spots on the opposite hand. Repeat on the other hand.

✈ Next, grab the left thumb with the thumb and index finger of the right hand. Gently pull it out with a rhythmic milking motion. Repeat on each finger of each hand.

✈ Place your right thumb on the palm of your left hand, and the other four fingers of your right hand around the back of the left hand, so that the index finger of your right hand rests against the base of the left index finger. Make circles into your palm with your right thumb. Move it all around the palm, stopping and spending more time in any areas that feel tight. Flip your left hand around, and do the same on the back of the hand. Make tiny circles around the bones near your wrist (carpal bones). Repeat on the other hand.

~ Legs ~

From other sections — #2, #4, #13.

#20 — Leg Extension

✈ Clear the luggage storage section in front of your feet. Extend your legs as much as you can. Point your toes and stretch your legs. Then flex your feet, bringing your toes back towards you and stretching the backs of your legs. Repeat several times.

✈ If you are seated in the first row (bulkhead seat) of the economy class, you may find yourself with a wall in front of you and enough space to extend your legs and touch the wall with your toes. If so, slowly extend your legs so that they are straight out in front of you and slightly below your hip level. Point your toes and press them against the wall in front of you. Then flex your feet, bringing your toes back towards you. Point and flex again. Make small tapping motions with your toes, alternating with the right and then the left foot, in quick rhythmic fashion. Then bend your knees and bring your feet back to the floor.

If you find yourself particularly prone to leg stiffness or poor circulation, you might want to request one of these seats. (The one drawback is that you cannot store carry-on luggage on the floor in front of you.) If you have varicose veins, you may want to wear support hose. If you have a nonbulkhead seat and have circulation problems in your legs, it can be helpful to rest your feet on your luggage in front of you.

#21 — Hamstring Stretches

Find an appropriate time to get up and walk up and down the aisle (not during meal or beverage service!). Stand in the aisle facing the outside of an aisle seat, or if there is room, stand behind the last seat. Place your hands on the edge of the seat, and place your right foot slightly in front of the left. Lunge forward, allowing your left heel to drop to the floor, and press your left hip forward, while moving your weight forward and back on the left leg. This will stretch out your left hamstring. Repeat on the other side. Then place your feet parallel and bounce from one foot to the other, alternating the transfer of weight and allowing each leg to stretch. Since you are transferring your weight from one leg to the other, this will also help your circulation.

~ Feet and Ankles ~

From other sections — #20, #21, #37.

#22 — Foot Stretch

With feet flat on the floor, lift the right heel, stretching the foot. Replace, and repeat on the left side. Then lift the toes of the right foot off the floor, flexing the foot. Replace, and repeat on the left. Repeat as much as you'd like, and finish by gently shaking each foot.

#23 — Arch Lift

Keeping your feet planted firmly on the floor, your toes and heels in place, lift just the arches. If your foot cramps, gently shake it out. This may be difficult at first, but it will get easier with time.

#24 — Piano Exercises for Your Toes

Again, keeping your feet flat on the floor, try to tap the sole of your shoe (or the floor, if you have removed your shoes) with each toe, one at a time, starting with the big toe and working your way to the pinky toe. Some toes may be easier than others. This is a really tricky one, so don't get discouraged if you have difficulty! It will come with practice.

#25 — Foot Self-Massage and Reflexology

For a brief explanation of Reflexology, see exercise #19.

✈ Remove your shoes and, with socks still on, rub all around the soles, ankles, and toes. Or better yet, if you feel comfortable doing so, remove your socks, apply lotion to each foot, and rub.

✈ Grab your foot with both hands, so that your thumbs rest on the top of your foot, and the remaining fingers of both hands are underneath the sole, with the fingers tips touching each other around the midline. Pull outward letting your fingers glide away from each other in smooth rhythmic strokes.

✈ If you have enough leg room, place the outside of your foot on the opposite knee. Wrap both hands around your foot, so that the thumbs rest on the middle of the sole, towards the pinky edge, and the remaining fingers rest on the top of the foot. Now rotate the hands in opposition, creating a rhythmic wringing-out motion (i.e., the right hand will move up and out while the left hand moves down and in).

✈ Start to rub all around the sole of your foot. Pay particular attention to any spot that feels sore, using even, rhythmic strokes. Avoid jabbing. Make small circles with your thumbs, and stroke gently with your knuckles moving side to side and up and down the surface of the foot. Pay particular attention to the inside border of each foot, along the arch.

✈ Make circles with your finger tips around the ankles.

> **Avoid using strong, direct pressure around the ankle and slightly above it on the inside of your leg if you are pregnant.** The reflexes to the reproductive organs lie in this region, and the application of intense pressure could upset the delicate balance in your body.

✈ Locate the crease at the base of your toes. Take your thumb and work your way around this general area (this area pertains to your neck, according to reflexology). Now start rubbing all around the base of the big toe, and continue in a straight line down the sole of the foot about an inch and a half (this area relates to your lungs). Now locate a major crease that crosses your sole about an inch below your toes. Locate the spot on this line that lies below your second toe. Press into this spot for a few seconds (this spot corresponds to your diaphragm, according to reflexology, and your kidneys, according to shiatsu). Next, find the spot on the base of the heel that is straight down from this point; press for a few seconds (this point also represents your kidneys, according to shiatsu, and your lower back, according to reflexology).

✦ If you are having a sinus headache, grab the tip of your second toe and squeeze.

✦ Take your knuckles, and gently roll up and down the length of the foot, and then back and forth in rows, starting at the base of the toes and working your way down towards the heel.

#26 — Ankle Rotation

Rotate your ankles in a circle. Start with them straight in front of you. Then, slowly and with control, move them so that the toes of the right foot move in a clockwise direction, while at the same time, the toes of the left foot move in a counterclockwise direction (i.e., circle outward). Continue the motion all the way around, making a complete circle. Then reverse this action, starting with the right foot moving in a counterclockwise direction, while the left foot moves in a clockwise direction (i.e., circle inward). Be aware of making a complete, even rotation. If you have weak ankles or a past sprain or injury, there is a tendency to exaggerate some parts of the circle and cheat others. If this is the case for you, pay particular attention to the part of the circle where your toes are facing outward away from the body. Make sure you don't neglect this part of the rotation. Also, if you have difficulty lifting both feet off the ground at once, do each foot separately.

~ Head and Neck ~

From other sections — # 10, #11, #37.

#27 — Neck Tilts

Be very passive and gentle in these exercises — no sudden jerks or bounces, as they are not effective and can actually cause injuries.

✈ Sitting upright, slowly drop your head forward, so that your chin is tucked in to your chest. Slowly and with control, bring your head back up, looking straight ahead. Gently drop it to the back. Then bring it back to the center. Do this two to three times.

✈ Slowly turn your head to the right side. Try to make it a pure turn without tilting, i.e., you should be looking to the side, not forward. That comes next! Slowly bring it back to center. Turn it to the left, and bring it back to center. Repeat this two to three times.

✈ Slowly tilt your head so that your right ear almost rests on your right shoulder. Stay there, and hold that position for a few seconds. Feel how it gives you a stretch on the left side of the neck. Do the same on the other side. Repeat two to three times.

#28 — Neck Stretch with Breathing

Sit straight up, facing forward. Take a deep breath and exhale. Repeat. On the next inhale, turn your head so you're looking to the right. On the exhale, gently lower your head so you're looking down at your shoulder. Inhale and lift your head. Exhale and face center. Repeat on the other side. Do this one slowly and gently, without forcing anything.

#29 — Neck and Back Stretch

Clasp your hands, place them behind your head at the place where your neck and head are joined, and slowly curl your chin into your chest. Think of your head as an extension of your spine. Again, be very passive; do not bounce. The idea is to let gravity take over. Make sure your head is really hanging, that you are not holding it up. If you can see what's in front of you in this position, you are not doing it correctly. While remaining curled down and keeping your chin tucked in, slowly turn your head to the right. Stay there for a few seconds and breathe deeply, feeling yourself releasing further. Keeping your chin tucked in, slowly turn your head back to center, and then turn slowly to the left. Hold for a few seconds and breathe, then slowly come back to center.

Keep your chin tucked in and continue to go lower, visualizing more and more links being added to your spine and the space between each link expanding. As long as it feels comfortable to do so, at each level, turn your head to the right, back to center, left, and back to center. Always bring your head back to the center position as you descend. You may discover a spot that feels particularly sore. Stay there a while and breathe deeply into that spot. When you've had enough, come up slowly and with control, rolling up starting at the base of the spine and working your way up. When you are upright, you can release your hands.

Now, without using your hands, tuck your chin into your chest, and slowly curl forward as far as you can, letting your head rest on your knees if you can. Stay there for a little while and breathe deeply. Again, come up slowly, curling your spine up from the bottom, lifting your head last. Be especially careful not to thrust your head forward while coming up if the seat in front of you is in the reclined position. Never jump up suddenly. This will undo all the good you've just done!

If you have persistent neck pain or an injury, you may want to bring an inflatable pillow. They are inexpensive and take up little room in your luggage, and also provide excellent neck support if you fall asleep.

#30 — Head Rolls

Note: the feasibility of doing this exercise is dependent on the height of the airplane seat, your height, and your flexibility. If you're fairly limber, experiment; if not, go on the next one!

If you are able to do this without too much discomfort, remove your shoes and bend up one leg, placing it on your seat, and then the other, so that you're kneeling on your seat, and then sit on your feet. This will allow you to sit even more erect than before. Allow your spine to elongate as much as possible. Now, lean your head back, so that the top of your seat supports the base of your skull. Gently roll your head so that your right ear touches the top of the seat. Bring it back to center, and then let your left ear touch the top of the seat. Continue this motion in a rhythmic fashion, letting your head gently roll from one side to the other. Don't try to control the motion with muscle exertion. It should be very passive and relaxed, and should feel very relaxing.

#31 — Scalp Massage

Scalp massage can relieve headaches and tension and increase circulation.

Make small circles all along the scalp, using the pads of the fingers. If you have a headache, stay in the spot where the pain is. Rub back and forth with short firm strokes. Trace the part of the head that runs parallel to and around the outside of the ears. You will feel four ridges running from the tops of the ears behind the hair line to a few inches above them. Press firmly in between the ridges, and rhythmically rub back and forth. Working these points usually relieves headaches.

~ Face and Eyes ~

From other sections — #2.

#32 — Monkey Face

You may prefer to wait do this one until after they have turned off the cabin lights (for reasons that will soon become apparent).

✦ Tighten your eyes into a ball, then your mouth, your lips, and the rest of your face. Make it as contracted as possible. Then completely release the tension.

✦ Move your jaw in a large circular motion, as though you were mouthing "yeow" in an exaggerated fashion. Repeat this two more times.

✦ Stick your tongue out of your mouth, drop it down, and stretch it out as far as it will comfortably go. Put it back in your mouth. Then stretch your eyes open wide as if you are startled, and relax. You can do these either separately or at the same time.

#33 — Eye Exercises

Your eyes will feel the effects of traveling. Lack of proper sleep, exposure to air pollution, and long hours staring at the computer screen all contribute to eye strain.

✦ To relieve this, begin by looking straight ahead. Without moving your head, slowly move your eyes to the right, then back to center, then to the left, and back to center. Then look up, center, down, and back to center.

✈ Move your eyes in a circle, starting to the right, then continuing up, to the left, down, and back to the right. Make it one smooth, continuous motion. Repeat two to three times. Reverse directions, beginning to the left, then traveling up, to the right, down, and back to the left. Repeat.

✈ Alternate focusing on something close and something far away.

✈ See exercise #35 for a visualization to relax the eyes.

#34 — Facial Massage and Acupressure

When we think of muscles, very few of us think of our face, but it is literally covered with delicate muscles, without which we could neither chew nor express our basic emotions. As our shoulders and backs bear the brunt of stress and strain, so do our faces. We "stiffen up our upper lip," "grin and bear it," "swallow our pride." Those of us who work at computers often experience eye strain and tension headaches. Most of the shiatsu meridians pass through the face and neck, so it is very therapeutic to apply pressure to various points on the face. Also, the sinuses are in the head, and if you apply pressure to the appropriate points, you can often get immediate relief from sinus headaches. As the air on planes is often stale and dry, these techniques may prove to be invaluable.

✈ Bend your elbows and bring your arms in front of you so that your palms are in front of your face. Now take the heels of both hands and place them next to one another at your hairline. Gently and slowly press them down your forehead. When you get to your eyes, be extremely gentle, and let your hands rotate. Let your wrists glide all the way to the outside of your face so that they brush against your ears. This can be very soothing for eye strain or general fatigue.

✦ Place each index finger on the outside of each brow at the temples. Gently trace the brows, moving towards the bridge of the nose. Continue down on either side of the nose, tracing the orbits (eye sockets), continuing the circle outward and back up to the temples. Follow the same pattern, making tiny, very gentle circles.

✦ Bring your thumbs together in the center of your forehead, at the hairline, so that the pads of your thumbs are touching your forehead. Gently press outward in the direction of your ears. Work your way down in rows. The last row should go across your eyebrows.

✦ Place your middle fingers at your temples. Make smooth circles. Now place your fingers at your jaws. Make circles there with several fingers at a time.

✦ Place your index fingers on either side at the center of the base of your skull at the point where your fingers sink in. Make circles, reversing direction. Take your thumbs and brush up and down from this area to about an inch above it. Now let your thumbs slide about a half an inch apart on each side. You should find a protrusion at the back of your head. This is the occipital ridge. You should feel another hollow on either side. Circle again with your fingers into these spaces. Now bring your hands lower and outward, to a point just under the bottom of your ears where you find another hollow. Circle your fingers once again.

There are many back and neck muscles which connect to the preceding areas. There are also many nerves in this region. Working these areas can relieve headaches, eye strain, neck and backaches, and sinus problems, so don't leave them out!

✦ With your right hand, grab your left shoulder and squeeze the muscle. Let go and grab and squeeze the area just above it. Work your way up the neck with this milking motion.

Face and Eyes

Do the same with your right shoulder and neck, using your left hand.

✈ Run your fingers across your eyebrows. You should notice a slight depression in the bone that goes around your eye (the orbit) toward the center, above the inner edge of your iris (diagram, point A). These are your frontal sinuses. Take your thumbs and press them firmly and steadily on this point on each side. Hold for a few seconds.

✈ Carefully run your thumbs straight down, about 1/8 of an inch below that point, so that they are resting up under the bone (B). This is a shiatsu point for headaches. Press at a 45 degree angle up and towards the back of your head. Hold for a few seconds. Leaving your thumbs gently resting up under the brows, place the remaining four fingers of each hand on your eyebrow. Gently grasp and squeeze the brow with your thumbs. The other fingers merely provide support.

✈ Slowly work your thumbs inward, and rub them gently up and down on the inner border of the orbits, slightly above the bridge of your nose (C). This is another headache relief area (the ethmoidal sinuses).

✈ Place your thumbs on the bottom of the orbits, about an inch below your irises (D). You should feel a slight depression in the bone. These are your maxillary sinuses. Press straight in towards the back of your head. Hold for a few seconds.

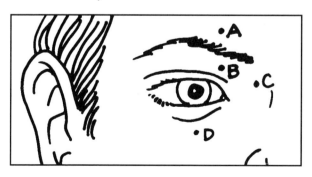

✈ Place your right index finger under your right nostril. With your left index finger, squeeze the nostril. Repeat on the other side. This will also clear your sinuses.

✈ Finally, place one thumb on top of the other. Place them in the roof of your mouth and press up. This will help move the many small bones that make up your sinuses and allow freer breathing.

A tip — If the altitude on the plane is bothering you and you feel pressure building up in your head, pinch your nose closed and blow out hard through your nose. Your ears will pop, and you should get some immediate relief.

~ VISUALIZATIONS

Visualizations can help to facilitate relaxation by engaging your mind in a beneficial way. Remember, you can also benefit by visualizing any of the other exercises in this book.

#35 — Inner Facial Glow

Close your eyes and imagine the muscles under your eyes getting wider and softer. Imagine soft light of any color you feel attracted to (white, green, or blue are best) surrounding your face, traveling under, above, and behind your eyes. Feel your face becoming as steady and serene as a Madonna, Buddha, or other image you may have seen in sculpture or painting that conveyed some form of calm, beautiful inner peace and strength. Or think of any experience you have had in your life that made you truly happy. Let yourself reexperience that happiness.

#36 — Visualizing Exercise

Visualize yourself doing your favorite sport or exercise, or one that you have always wanted to try. Have fun with it!

#37 — Visualizations for Good Posture and More Efficient Movement Patterns

The body is designed in such a way that there are ideal ways of aligning it efficiently to use the bones and skeletal muscles for optimum support. Most of us, unfortunately, have postural habits which put strain on certain muscles and underuse others. The result is often chronic pain or fatigue. To rectify this problem, one solution would be to perform corrective exercises. Another alternative is to imagine or visualize certain movements occurring in one's body while remaining still. Sitting in an airplane can be an ideal setting to experiment with these exercises for several reasons. 1) You're stuck in your seat anyway. It will give you something to do. 2) Focusing on your body in a therapeutic way may relieve some discomfort and help you improve your alignment, allowing you to feel more comfortable in your body. 3) If you're uncomfortable doing some of the more active exercises, visualizations can be performed without anyone around you knowing that you're doing them. And 4) by concentrating on these somatic images, your mind will begin to relax.

Lulu Sweigard*, a movement educator and researcher in kinesiology, developed "ideokinesis," a method for realigning the skeletal structure to produce better alignment and more efficient movement patterns. She cites nine "lines of movement," which, when imagined correctly and consistency,

*Adapted with permission from *Human Movement Potential: Its Ideokinetic Facilitation*, by Lulu E. Sweigard. University Press of America, 1988. Harper & Row, Publishers, Inc., 1974.

can actually produce improved carriage and flexibility. I will now describe each line of movement and the corresponding exercises she suggests, which can be done in the seated position to produce a more harmonious use of the body. Please remember, these are mental exercises; do nothing with your body other than sit upright, and imagine the movements as vividly as you can.

✦ First of all, imagine your spine as an upright rod on which your head rests. There is a crosswise rod at the shoulder level on which a coat hangs. Try to sit on your "sits bones" and not the back of your pelvis or your tailbone.

✦ The first line of movement releases tightness of the back muscles, particularly the lower or lumbar region. You should imagine your torso as an ice cream sandwich, in a vertical position, with a back slice of chocolate, a middle ice cream filling, and a front slice of chocolate. See the back slice sliding downward.

✦ The second line of movement releases the muscles on the back of the pelvis, which, when contracted, can restrict hip flexion. Imagine the pelvis as a toy accordion, with handles on either side and vertical pleats on the back. Watch the accordion being opened wide in the back to smooth out all the pleats. Or see the pelvis as a circular shower curtain ring with two hanging curtains on the back of the rim. See the curtains separating at the center in the back and moving outward towards the front.

✦ The third line of movement helps the thigh bone align itself deep within the center of the hip socket and allows the surrounding muscles to work efficiently. Imagine a rod the diameter of a broomstick going from the center of the knee deep into the center of the thigh socket. Most people tend to aim the hip end of the stick to the outside of the socket and not deep enough inside the socket. Visualize the stick moving both closer into the center and deeper within. Imagine that there is an uncooked bagel on some point on this pole (A). The dough is falling apart on the inner rim of the bagel. Watch it being molded to firm up the inside, making sure that it doesn't sag downward against the stick (B). Then watch the bagel sliding carefully and slowly towards the inside of the socket, making sure that the bagel stays firm, that the inside does not fall apart, and that the inside surface moves at the same rate as the outside surface.

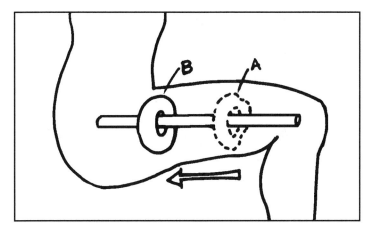

✈ The fourth line of movement releases tension in the chest and thoracic area of the back, allowing a more flexible rib cage and freer breathing. Visualize the rib cage inside the shoulders as a large fat prune, extending from the base of the neck to the level of the lowest ribs. Watch it wrinkle all over to shrink away from the shoulders towards the center, until its circumference is reduced to that of a broomstick.

✈ The fifth line of movement produces better pelvic alignment and aids the other lines of movement. Imagine the pelvis as a basketball with a vertical opening at the center-front of the pelvis that must be laced together. Watch the sides of the opening being pulled together as the lacing proceeds from the bottom upward.

✈ The sixth line of movement aids in better alignment and use of the foot and ankle in walking. Imagine you are wearing flippers which are stuck in mud. Watch the foot being pulled out of the mud, first heels, and then the toes.

✈ The seventh line of movement also helps to realign the pelvis. Imagine the pelvis as the rim of an ice cream cone. It tips down in front so that the scoop of ice cream bulges towards the front, as thought it were pressing on the inside of your belly, and places pressure against the mid-front of the rim of the cone (A). Watch the front rim of the cone moving up to a level position to allow the scoop of ice cream to fall back into place within the rim. Finally, watch a cherry at the level of the bottom of the rib cage moving forward to the center top of the ice cream scoop. (B)

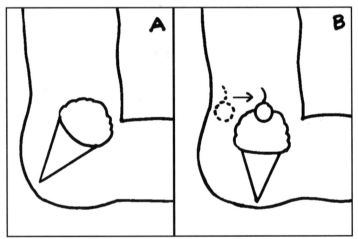

✈ The eighth line of movement helps to align the head in relation to the neck. Imagine a cap on the back of the head. Watch it sliding over the top of the head to reach the level of the eyebrows.

✈ The ninth line of movement lengthens the spine upward. Imagine that your neck is growing like an Alice-in-Wonderland neck to raise the head higher and higher. It is very pliable, but also very strong.

~ SUGGESTED ROUTINES ~

While you can easily mix and match the preceding exercises to suit your personal needs and preferences, these routines will help you to get started.

Routine 1

#1 — Sitting Up Straight
#3 — Spinal Twist
#6 — Arm Stretches
#8 — Shoulder Lifts and
   Drops
#12 — Pelvic Tilts
#13 — Leg Isometrics
#17 — Wrist and Hand
   Release
#21 — Hamstring Stretches
#22 — Foot Stretch
#27 — Neck Tilts

#33 — Eye Exercises
#36 — Visualizing Exercise

Routine 2

#2 — Wake-up
#5 — Waist Lengthener
#7 — Breathing
#9 — Shoulder Rolls
#10 — Neck and Shoulder
   Release
#14 — Rib Cage Isolations
#16 — Hand Grip and
   Pectoral Strengthener
#4 — Leg and Hip Stretch
#26 — Ankle Rotation
#29 — Neck and Back
   Stretch
#32 — Monkey Face
#35 — Inner Facial Glow

Self-Massage Routine

#31 — Scalp Massage
#34 — Facial Massage and Acupressure
#18 — Neck, Shoulder, and Arm Self-Massage
#19 — Hand Self-Massage and Reflexology
#25 — Foot Self-Massage and Reflexology

You may want to try one of the following to alleviate a particular discomfort:

Stiffness or sluggishness — General Warm-Up section.
Circulation — #2, #20, #21, any of the self-massage exercises.
Lower back pain — #12, #13.
Headache or sinus — #19, #25, #27, #31, #34.

Making Your Trip More Comfortable

Along with the discomfort that comes from being confined to your seat for a long period of time, travel often has other side effects. While this section doesn't cover every side effect or every remedy, it will cover many of the more common effects and a smorgasbord of remedies that you can choose from.

Some over-the-counter remedies and dietary changes are suggested. Also featured are what are now called alternative remedies, including vitamins, herbs, homeopathy, and Bach Flower Remedies. These are generally available in health food stores and some pharmacies. If you find that any of these appeal to you, I would suggest that you research them further, or try them out and see which ones work best for you. Many books are available, including those listed at the back of this book, and you might enjoy exploring your local health food store.

> When using any of the remedies in this book, consult the labels for special instructions.
>
> If you have a medical condition or are taking any medication, or are pregnant or nursing, it is strongly recommended that you not try any of these remedies before consulting your health professional.
>
> When dealing with children, use moderation in all remedies.

General Comfort

✈ Store carry-ons overhead to give more leg room, or use them to prop your feet up.

✈ Dress in loose, comfortable clothing and shoes.

✈ Pack the following items in a carry-on: inflatable neck pillow, sleep mask, ear plugs, slippers, Walkman, bottled spring water, wash-n-dries (for face and hands), healthy snacks, hand lotion, peppermint foot lotion, as well as any of the remedies in this section that you anticipate needing. Generally, small pillows and blankets are available on the plane.

✈ For the hotel room, you might want to pack a hot water bottle or heating pad. Foot soaks, such as those from Dr. Scholl's or Johnson's, are excellent for sore feet after a day of walking, and can even be used as bath salts for the entire body.

Aromatherapy. This is the use of essential oils to heal ailments or alter your mood in a safe, gentle way. Although many have the same names as herbs, the form is different. Consult an aromatherapy book for more specific information, or better yet, try them out to see what appeals to you. They generally come in small bottles that can be kept in a purse or pocket for easy accessibility.

✈ Makes you feel good: apple, damiana (feeling of well being), gardenia, geranium, lilac, lily, magnolia, narcissus, sweet pea, water lily, wood aloe.

✈ Promotes calm or relaxation: catnip, lavender (also good for headaches), rue.

✈ Promotes restful sleep: bergamot, celery, chamomile, hops, jasmine, marjoram.

Herbs. Herbs are readily available in health food stores and many pharmacies.

✈ Relaxant, calming, good for sleep: catnip tea (relaxant), chamomile (relaxing), gotu kola, hops, jasmine, kava kava, motherwort, orange flowers tea, passion flower, St. John's wort, skullcap, valerian.

✈ Circulation: bilberry tea (also good for the eyes), butcher's broom, gingko biloba, gotu kola, hawthorne berries.

✈ Makes you feel good: damiana.

While at the Airport

Often travelers experience muscle soreness and related physical problems as a result of having carried heavy luggage around the airport prior to, as well as after, the flight. To ease this problem, use a luggage cart whenever possible. If you must carry your bags, try to distribute the weight evenly. Don't put four bags on your right shoulder and one on the left; try to balance them, no matter how awkward this may feel. If you bend over to lift a suitcase from the floor, hold your stomach in, curl your pelvis under, and curl your back up, using your legs. Don't rise up by arching your lower back or thrusting your chest forward. If you are on a long line, put your luggage down; don't balance it on your shoulders any longer than you have to.

If you're traveling with a companion, take turns having someone sit with the luggage while the other person walks around the airport. Find a private place, such as a rest room stall, and do some shoulder rolls to release the tension. While sitting, twist at the waist to each side to stretch your lower back. If you have the space (sitting or standing), curl your chin into your chest and slowly curl down so that your palms approach or touch the floor. Release your head, and shake out your head, neck, and shoulders. Slowly come up, starting at the base of the spine and curling up sequentially, vertebrae by vertebrae, to an upright position.

Jet Lag

Jet lag is a cluster of uncomfortable symptoms experienced by people who travel rapidly across several time zones. Its severity is determined by the number of time zones crossed during the flight, and only occurs when one travels across time zones from either east to west or west to east, and never from north to south or the reverse. Jet lag is a recent phenomenon experienced by travelers since the introduction of air travel and is caused by the body's inability to adjust its inner clock to rapid changes in time. Your circadian rhythms are set by exposure to light and the hormonal rhythms of melatonin, which is produced during the night by the pineal gland. The symptoms of jet lag include disorientation, memory loss, grogginess, irritability, and difficulty in falling asleep or waking up at the appropriate time. It is said that it takes the body one full day for every hour difference in time, and it is usually more difficult for most people to adjust when traveling eastward, as it is unnatural to fall asleep earlier than one is accustomed to. It can be particularly trying for business travelers who must appear alert and follow the local schedule.

Melatonin. Several books have recently come out singing the praises of melatonin, which has found to be effective in treating various conditions, including jet lag. Two of these books include *The New York Times* best seller, *The Melatonin Miracle,* by Pierpaoli, Regelson, and Coleman, and *Melatonin: Your Body's Newest Wonder Drug,* by Reiter and Robinson. Most proponents of melatonin, including the authors of these two books, recommend ingesting three to five milligrams within an hour before retiring upon arrival at your destination. They emphatically recommend only taking it at night.

But in an article in *The New York Times*, Jane Brody cites contradictory advice from Dr. Alfred Lewy, an authority on circadian rhythms at the Oregon Health Sciences University in Portland. According to Dr. Lewy, if one is traveling west, one should take melatonin in the morning, and if one is traveling east, it is best to take it in the afternoon. For example, Dr. Lewy suggested that when traveling from Pacific to Eastern time, one should ingest melatonin at 2 PM the day before traveling, then take it the same time on the traveling day, and at 5 PM on the first day on the east coast. This will push the body clock forward, so that one could fall asleep at night and wake up in the morning, Eastern time. When one makes the reverse trip, one should take melatonin upon awakening all three days. This will have the effect of delaying the dawn and allowing you to go to bed later and awaken later.

Dr. Lewy cautions that taking melatonin at the wrong time can actually *induce* jet lag, that current doses are too high, and that more research needs to be done. Indeed, even on the bottle of melatonin I obtained in a health food store, the following contraindications were listed: pregnant or lactating women, children and teenagers, those with autoimmune diseases, diabetes, depressive disorders, epilepsy, and leukemia.

Yet another point of view was expressed in a *Newsweek* article by Dr. Ray Sahelian, a Los Angeles physician and the author of *Melatonin: Nature's Sleeping Pill,* who advises waiting until you reach your destination, and then taking melatonin at bed time, one milligram for every time zone you've crossed, up to 10 to 12 milligrams.

The use of melatonin is still in the experimental stage, and caution is advised. Side effects, such as nightmares, have been noted. At this time, Reiter and Robinson suggest that the following avoid melatonin: pregnant and nursing women and those trying to conceive, people with severe allergies or autoimmune diseases, people with immune system cancers such as lymphoma or leukemia, and healthy children (who already produce sufficient amounts). Consult with your doctor before using. If you'd like to do your own research, the books mentioned here are listed at the end of this book.

Melatonin: the natural way. Based on the same research, there is another, and perhaps safer, method to alter melatonin levels in our body. According to an article in *The New York Times* by Daniel Goleman, Dr. Lewy demonstrated in a 1980 study that exposure to light suppresses the production of melatonin, while darkness stimulates its production. Scientists at the National Institute of Mental Health were able to pinpoint the exact time when the eyes are exposed to bright light. They discovered that for the average person, 4 AM was a kind of threshold; exposure to light just prior to this point delays circadian rhythms, causing one to want to retire earlier than usual, and conversely, exposure to light immediately after 4 AM causes one to want to stay up later than usual. By altering the times that you are exposed to darkness or light, you can manipulate the environmental cues, which in turn triggers your circadian rhythms. Exposure to bright light on either side of this threshold apparently brings the strongest results.

Mr. Goleman recommends a book, *How to Beat Jet Lag*, by Dan Oren, which contains textual information, an eye mask, shades, and a table instructing one on how many time zones one may be crossing for various destinations and, therefore, the best time to expose one's eyes to darkness or light. One can control the exposure to light or darkness on a plane by using the sunglasses and eye shades or looking out the window. At times, because of the patterns of the sun in the direction in which you are traveling, it may be advantageous to request either a window or an aisle seat. Frequent fliers may even consider gazing into a flashlight or investing in a small light box when exposure to natural light is difficult.

Mr. Goleman gave an example of this technique with his trip from Newark to Copenhagen. He put sunglasses on at

10 PM Newark (Eastern Standard) time and didn't remove them until 10 AM Eastern Standard Time. To expose his eyes to light at the appropriate time, he looked out the plane window at bright northern sunlight. He has found these methods to be greatly effective in reducing the effects and duration of jet lag. But Mr. Oren and his colleagues caution that these methods will be of no avail for trips that last fewer than four days.

Foods. Eat brown rice or other complex carbohydrates such as pasta, bread, and potatoes. Avoid excess salt, sugar, and dairy.

✈ Do not smoke, and avoid second hand smoke in the airport; the toxins can stay in your system for several hours.

Vitamins and supplements. Take Ester C with bioflavonoids, B-complex, folic acid, B-12, and brewers yeast before the flight.

✈ According to *Healthy Healing: An Alternative Healing Reference*, by Linda G. Rector-Page, it is advisable to try Tyrosine 500 mg, 2-3 a day, a few days before the trip and during the trip as needed, raw pituitary extract twice a day for 8 days before traveling, and homeopathic Highland's *Calms Forté* as needed.

Herbs. Men may find it helpful to ingest ginseng before and during the trip. Women should avoid it, because it is too harsh for the female system. They can take dong quai, but only 3 to 5 days after their period, and even then, it should be used with some caution, because it can cause dehydration in some women.

Homeopathic Remedies. Homeopathy is a form of medicinal treatment developed by Samuel Hahnemann, a German doctor and chemist, in the eighteenth century. It is becoming popular again today because of its effectiveness and lack of toxic side effects. Homeopathic remedies are taken sublingually (dissolved under the tongue). You can also dissolve two pellets of each remedy in water and sip the water. (They dissolve more easily if the water is warm; you might find it easy to get a cup of hot water from the flight attendant, dissolve the pellets, and let it cool.)

When taking homeopathic remedies, you should avoid peppermint (including toothpaste), caffeine, alcohol, tobacco, and spicy foods for at least one hour before and after, if not completely. (Mint-free toothpaste is available in many health food stores.)

✦ Starting three days before your flight, take four pellets of Arnica twice a day for two days. Then, the day before the flight, the day of the flight, and the day after the flight, take four pellets three times a day. Repeat for the return trip. An alternative regimen is to take one 30x tablet every hour while on the plane.

✦ You can also take Nux Vomica to relieve some of the symptoms of jet lag, such as fatigue, insomnia, and upset stomach. Check your health food store or pharmacy for other homeopathic remedies that might be appropriate for you.

Dehydration

The dry air in an airplane cabin tends to cause dehydration, and jet lag is greatly exacerbated by dehydration. Drink lots of water before, during, and after the flight, even if you don't feel particularly thirsty; if you don't, you may well suffer for it the next day. I recommend bringing a large bottle of water with you and sipping it slowly throughout the flight, rather than gulping it all at once. Or bring along a sports drink, such as *Recharge* or *Gatorade*, to replenish your trace minerals, including potassium. Never drink alcohol on a plane even if they give it away! Try to avoid excessive amounts of salt, sugar, or dairy. When you arrive, try to eat at local meal times. This will also assist your body's adjustment.

Motion Sickness

Motion sickness is caused by an inner ear imbalance. The deaf do not get it, and women are more likely to suffer from this condition than men. Following are various methods you can choose from to alleviate motion sickness.

Foods. Chew gum or suck on a candy for take-offs and landings.

✈ Eat crackers or pretzels, drink carbonated water, peppermint tea, or ginger ale to settle your stomach. (Do not drink peppermint tea if taking homeopathics, as it is an antidote and will counteract the benefits). On short commuter flights, eat the snack the airline gives you, even if you are not hungry. Even a few cookies or pretzels will absorb excess gas and settle your stomach.

Vitamins and supplements. Take 500 milligrams of magnesium (a nerve tonic) one hour before the trip, and 100 mg of vitamin B6 one hour before the trip and again two hours later (to relieve nausea).

✈ Take vitamin B1 and 500 mg of thiamine before departure.

Herbs. If you are experiencing headaches, nausea, dizziness, lack of appetite, excess salivation, cold sweats, sleepiness, or vomiting due to travel motion, take *Motion Mate (TRVL)* from Nature's Way. It contains ginger root, meadowsweet, peppermint, red raspberry, and hyssop.

✈ Take activated charcoal tablets to absorb excess acids, and ginkgo biloba extract drops before and during the flight for inner ear balance.

✈ Take two to three ginger capsules an hour before traveling, and as needed throughout the trip.

✈ Take basil or anise.

Homeopathy. Try Borax, Cocculus Indicus, Nux Vomica, or Tabacum, or one of the following combinations: Hyland's *Motion Sickness* (Nux Vomica, Tabacum, Petroleum, Cocculus Indicus) or Dolisos' *Travel Sickness* (Belladonna, Cocculus Indicus, Colchicum, Ipecacuanha, Nux Vomica, Petroleum, Tabacum).

Self-massage. If you are feeling queasy, place one hand on top of the other and gently rest them just under the rib cage. Then lower them so that they rest over the navel area. Bend the fingers of the underneath hand into a fist while keeping the other hand extended, and press gently inward for firmer pressure. Rub the underpad of the fourth toe, or of the ring finger, to effect inner ear balance.

Other remedies. Don't read or look at a computer screen if you are feeling queasy. Close your eyes and listen to some relaxing music on a Walkman.

✈ Purchase Sea Bands in a drugstore or health food store. They are elastic bracelets that press on an acupuncture point on the inside of the wrists, which is effective in treating nausea. If you are not able to purchase them, you can press the point with your other hand. It is on the palm side of your arm about two fingers width up from the wrist crease, in between the two tendons. Press hard and directly for several seconds three times.

Upset Stomach

Foods. Bananas, cooked rice, peppermint tea, papaya (or papaya enzyme tablets).

✈ For nausea: warm and salty bullion, Gatorade. (See section on Motion Sickness.)

✈ Avoid: coffee with or without caffeine, fried and salted foods, carbonated beverages, fruit juice.

Homeopathy. Nux Vomica.

Herbs. For gas: bay leaves, cardamom, ginger, garlic, peppermint.

Diarrhea

Over-the-counter remedies. *Immodium* is highly recommended, especially when traveling in the Third World or anywhere that it may be difficult to find Western medicine. For milder cases, *Pepto-Bismol* or *Kaopectate* is fine.

Foods. Blackcurrant tea, blueberries, yogurt with live cultures, honey, rice, soy milk or soy beans, toast, chocolate. Follow the BRAT diet (bananas, rice, applesauce, and toast).

✈ Avoid: apple juice (especially children), coffee, wheat bran, most fruits and vegetables, salads, milk, sugar, sorbitol (a sugar substitute), beans.

✈ Drink only bottled beverages (carbonated is better than flat). Try chamomile tea (*manzanilla* in Spanish). Avoid unpasteurized dairy products, tap water, ice cubes, food from street vendors. When traveling in the Third World, eat only foods you can peel, boil, or that come from a sealed bottle. If you need to wash fruits or vegetables, boil the water first. You can also bring water purification tablets, available in sporting goods stores.

Herbs. A friend of mine traveled extensively throughout India and never got sick. He attributes it to taking a garlic pill before every meal.

Constipation

Foods. Wheat bran, barley, prunes or prune juice, dried beans, high fiber fruits and vegetables (carrots, cabbages, apples), other fruits and vegetables (especially peas, beans, nuts, dried fruits and berries, leafy vegetables like spinach, apples, oranges, prunes, figs, dates), oats, barley, kelp, coarse wheat bran, rice bran, whole wheat bread, coffee, lots of fluids.

✈ Avoid: milk.

Herbs. Alfalfa, apple, cascara sagrada (also called buckthorn), damiana, olive oil, psyllium, licorice tea, sarsparilla tea.

Insomnia

If you have trouble sleeping on a long flight, or when you reach your destination, try one of the following:

Homeopathic: Aconite, Coffea, Ignatia, Nux Vomica, or one of the following combinations: *Calms Forté* from Hyland (contains Passion Flower, Oat, Hops, Chamomile, Calcium Phosphate, Iron Phosphate, Potassium Phosphate, Sodium Phosphate, Magnesium Phosphate), *Insomnia & Anxiety* from Dolisos (Avena sativa, Chamomilla, Humulus lup., Passiflora, Coffea cruda, Ignatia), or *Insomnia Relief* from Homeolab USA (Passiflora incarnata, Valeriana officinale, Avena sativa, Cuprum aceticum, Hyoscyamus niger).

Herbs: Hops, jamaica dogwood, kava kava, lavender, lime blossom (safe for children), motherwort, passionflower, skullcap, and valerian. Many of these are available as capsules or tinctures (liquid), but are particularly effective in tincture form.

Aromatherapy: Clary sage.

Alertness and Energy

Herbs. According to Earl Mindell's *Herb Bible*, take suma, basil, borage tea (a pick-me up tonic), or guarana (stimulating effect, to fight fatigue). Men may try ginseng (it is too harsh for women, who may try dong quai, but only several days after their period, and it should be used with caution as it can cause dehydration in some women).

Aromatherapy. Benzoin, bergamot mint, black pepper, camphor, carnation, cinnamon, ginger lemon, lime nutmeg, orange, pennyroyal (not for pregnant women), saffron.

Sinus Problems

One of the unpleasant realities of air travel is that the air in the cabin is often stale and dry, which can lead to sinus problems. If you have these tendencies, and either feel uncomfortable performing the acupressure points (exercise #34) or find they are insufficient to alleviate the problem, I have several suggestions.

Over-the-counter. Take *Seldane* or a similar sinus medication one hour before landing.

Herbs. Drink *Breathe Easy*, a tea put out by Traditional Medicinals. Since the main ingredient in the tea is the herb ephedra, or ma huang, which is a stimulant, it is recommended that you do not consume this before bedtime. (Please note: Although, some forms of ephedra were recently taken off the market, when used in moderation, it should be perfectly safe. Any substance when taken in megadoses can be harmful, but the amount in a tea bag is minimal, and I have personally found this herb to be very therapeutic for myself and others. However, as with any herb or drug, if you have any side effects, discontinue use.)

Other remedies. If your have persistent sinus problems, or suffer from dehydration, and your job requires frequent travel and a lot of public speaking or vocal performance after plane trips, you might consider investing in a Kaz *TheraSteam*, a personal steam inhaler favored by professional singers, who cannot afford to have a dry throat and nasal passages. It is 7½ inches high, weighs less than a pound, and has its own travel bag for an additional fee. If you cannot find this item in a store or mail order catalogue, you can order the inhaler from Kaz directly for $49.95, and the travel bag for an additional $9.99, by calling 1-800-477-0457.

Fear of Flying

According to Farrol S. Kahn, author of *Why Flying Endangers Your Health**, fear of flying is extremely common, is often related to an inborn fear of both heights and falling, and can be overcome. In fact, in the early days of commercial flying, when cabin conditions were much more rustic than they are today and half the passengers got air sick, Steve Simpson, the president of United Airlines' San Francisco Office, was inspired to hire female nurses to calm the passengers down, look after their needs, and distract them from the discomforts of flying. Thus the concept of the modern stewardess was born!

Kahn recommends consulting an aviation medical expert to ensure that a potential health risk is not the source of your anxiety. If you are a true aerophobic, meaning that the fear is overpowering to the point that you are too frightened to fly, behavior modification therapy may help you slowly desensitize from this fear. If your level of fear is less overwhelming, but you are experiencing symptoms such as anxiety, insomnia,

---

*Adapted with permission from *Why Flying Endangers Your Health:Hidden Health Hazards of Air Travel*, by Farrol S. Kahn. Aurora Press, 1992.

---

hyperventilation, indigestion, or faintness before or during the flight, you may want to take relaxed-flying seminars, which most airlines run. You may be surprised to learn they are often attended by frequent fliers!

Kahn also cites the following health conditions which might make flying contraindicated: "In general, an unfit passenger is anyone who has a disease that impairs the heart's output, the lungs' ability to oxygenate the blood, the flow of blood through the circulatory system, the blood's oxygen-carrying capacity, or has blood that might clot readily. [If you have] a high risk condition, check with your M.D. . . ." Also included are those who have had recent surgery, and alcoholics with a history of delirium or Korasakoff's syndrome. Pregnant women in either the first or last trimester should consult their doctor before flying.

Homeopathy. Argentum Nitricum (Argent. nit.) for anxieties, fears, and phobias.

Bach Flower Remedies. This series of flower essences was developed by Dr. Edward Bach in the 1930's to alleviate a wide range of emotional conditions. There are 38, plus Rescue Remedy, and the choice of remedy is based on your specific fears. Following are some suggestions. Consult a practitioner or book for information on the complete line. *Bach Flower Therapy*, by Mechthild Scheffer, is an excellent resource.

Suggested Bach remedies for fear of flying are: Aspen (vague, unknown fears; anxiety and apprehension), Cherry Plum (fear of losing control of thoughts and actions), Mimulus (fear of known things: heights, the dark, being alone, etc.), Rock Rose (terror, extreme fright and panic; nightmares), Rescue Remedy (gentle, calming, and stabilizing in a variety of stressful situations).

When You Arrive

If this has been a long flight, or you are in a different climate or altitude than you are used to, pace yourself. If possible, take the first two days to adjust. Plan few activities and allow for a lot of rest. Be sure to continue to drink a lot of water. If you are arriving in daylight, try to get outside immediately, to help reset your biological clock. Take a walk outside to feel grounded.

If you're on a business trip with a tight schedule, try to take a few minutes to relax, take a shower, or perhaps do a few of the exercises on pages 50-51 before you run to your meeting. Carry bottled water in your briefcase, and don't skip meals.

✈ Complex carbohydrates are recommended for high altitudes.

✈ If you are having difficulty staying awake when you need to, eat light, spicy meals and fruit.

✈ If you are having difficulty sleeping, eat cheese, miso soup with scallions, and bland food, and drink calming teas such as chamomile. (You may need to carry your own tea bags as well as a heating element with the appropriate currency.) Bring the tissue salt called "insomnia" with you or Highland's *Calms Forté* if you have this tendency. (Tissue salts are inorganic salts essential to the body, prepared in homeopathic form, and available in health food stores.)

✈ If the stress and strain of traveling leaves you with muscle cramps, rub *Tiger Balm* or Vicks *Vaporub* into the spot. Apply a hot water bottle or heating pad (moist is better than dry) for brief periods. (Do not sleep with a heating pad on! It can be harmful to your body and cause a fire.) Do not sleep in the nude (i.e., if you have a knot in your shoulder, wear a shirt or nightgown; if it is in your leg, wear pajama bottoms; and if it is in your neck, sleep with either a scarf around your neck or a turtleneck). The idea is to keep the area warm. The *Tiger Balm* brings blood to the area, and the clothing will keep the area warm, as well as protect you from drafts.

✈ If at all possible, try to get a professional massage. It will calm your nerves, improve your circulation, work out muscle aches, and make it easier to sleep at night. I've been told that Virgin Atlantic offers on-board mini-chair massages on their London-New York flights, and that they have a lounge at Heathrow where they offer hour-long, full-body table massages. Many hotels have massage therapists on call or on staff at their health clubs, or through the concierge. If you're a budget traveler, try staying at a Y instead of a bargain hotel. The price of your room will include free access to their gym and pool. Many Y's have huge facilities with a wide array of classes and equipment. Many offer massage as well. Even if you choose to stay elsewhere, you can use the facilities for a small daily fee, or they may be available to you free of charge if you are a member of a Y in another city.

✈ If your trip involves a lot of walking, pick up some peppermint foot lotion. At the end of each day, rub it vigorously on your feet and legs. Then elevate your legs. If a tub or basin is available, first soak your feet using a foot soak, such as Dr. Scholl's or Johnson's. You can also use these in the tub to soak your entire body.

Exercises You Can Do In Your Hotel Room

Now that you have more space to work with, here are a few exercises you can do to loosen up after your trip.

▰ Lie on the floor. Tuck your knees in to your chest. Grab them with your hands and rock your spine gently back and forth.

▰ Sit straight on the floor with your legs extended in front of you. Hang your head over and round your back so that your head approaches your knees. If you're flexible enough, let your head touch your knees. If not, drop it wherever you are, and let it be very passive and heavy. Take a deep breath and let it out. Then circle your ankles in each direction. Curl up slowly.

▰ Bring the soles of your feet together. Roll back on your sit bones and let your head passively drop forward. Move the area under your rib cage in a circle, first clockwise, then counterclockwise, letting your pelvis rock back and forth in a circular motion.

▰ Sitting straight up, spread your legs wide apart with your knees facing up to the ceiling. Drop your head forward. Slowly turn your body until it's over your right leg, and drop your head to your knee. Rest there. Repeat on the left. Then come back to center and drop forward. Roll up slowly.

▰ Half Sit-ups. Lie on your back with your knees bent and your feet flat on the floor. Place your hands behind your head, protecting and supporting your neck. Slowly curl up to a sitting position, exhaling as your curl up. Then gently lie back, inhaling. If you are unable to come to a full sitting position, simply do "stomach crunches," bringing your head and shoulders up as far as you can, using your stomach muscles.

Repeat several times. You can vary this by reaching for the opposite knee with your elbow.

▬ Kneeling on your hands and knees, relax your back. Then tighten your stomach muscles and arch your back. Relax. Repeat several times.

▬ The Plough. If you are flexible, lie on your back, extend your legs out and bring them up and over your head so that your feet rest on the ground above your head. Hold for a few seconds, or for as long as feels comfortable.

▬ Shoulder Stand. If you are very limber, lie on your back, throw your legs over your head, support your hips with your arms, and lift your legs in the air. Let one leg drop forward and the other one drop back. Reverse. Note: It is inadvisable for menstruating women to do this.

▬ Standing up, clasp your hands together, extend your arms downward, and slowly roll your head and spine down towards the floor, curling down from the top vertebrae. Rest there and breathe. When you're ready to come up, slowly curl up from the bottom of the spine, vertebrae by vertebrae, until your head comes up. Breathe.

▬ Release your hands, letting them fall to your sides. Drop to your right side, allowing your torso to bend from the waist, and then to the left. Repeat a few times.

▬ With your feet wide apart, reach your left arm down, out, up, and around, lifting it over your head to the right. Bend at the waist and allow your right knee to bend. If you need to, support yourself by placing your right hand on your thigh. Let your arm follow the same path back to your side and come back to a standing position. Repeat on the other side.

You can also do many of the exercises listed in the previous sections. Among them are: #3, #5, #8, #14, #20, #28, and #30.

SUGGESTED READING

Balch, James F., M.D., and Balch, Phyllis A., C.N.C. *Prescription for Nutritional Healing: A Practical A-Z Reference To Drug-Free Remedies Using Vitamins, Minerals, Herbs & Food Supplements*, Avery Publishing Group, 1990.

Brody, Jane. "Personal Health: Debate Aside, Melatonin Can Reset the Body's Clock," *The New York Times*, Wednesday, September 27, 1995, Section C, National Desk, p. 9.

Carper, Jean. *The Food Pharmacy*, Bantam Books, 1988.

Carper, Jean. *Food — Your Miracle Medicine*, HarperCollins, 1993.

Cowley, Geoffrey. "Melatonin Mania," *Newsweek*, November 6, 1995.

Goleman, Daniel. "Easing Jet Lag by Resetting the Body Clock," *The New York Times*, Sunday, August 13, 1995, Section 5, Travel Desk, p.18.

Hoffman, David. *An Herbal Guide to Stress Relief*, Healing Arts Press, 1991.

Kahn, Farrol S. *Why Flying Endangers Your Health: Hidden Health Hazards of Air Travel*, Aurora Press, 1992.

Lockie, Dr. Andrew, and Geddes, Dr. Nicola. *The Complete Guide to Homeopathy: The Principles & Practice of Treatment*, Dorling Kindersley, 1995.

Mindell, Earl. *Earl Mindell's Herb Bible*, Simon & Schuster/ Fireside, 1992.

Norman, Laura, with Cowan, Thomas. *Feet First: A Guide to Foot Reflexology*, Simon & Shuster,1988.

Ohashi, Wataru. *Do it Yourself Shiatsu: How to Perform the Ancient Japanese Art of Acupuncture Without Needles*, E.P. Dutton, 1976.

Oren, Dan, M.D. *How to Beat Jet Lag: A Practical Guide for Air Travelers*, Henry Holt and Co., 1993.

Pierpaoli, Walter, M.D., Ph.D., and Regelson, William, M.D., with Coleman, Carol. *The Melatonin Miracle*, Simon and Shuster, 1995.

Rector-Page, Linda G., R.N. *Healthy Healing: An Alternative Healing Reference*, Healthy Healing Publication, 1992.

Reiter, Russel J., Ph.D., and Robinson, Jo. *Melatonin: Your Body's Natural Wonder Drug*, Bantam Books, 1995.

Rick, Stephanie. *The Reflexology Workout: Hand & Foot Massage for Super Health & Rejuvenation*, Harmony Books, 1986.

Sahelian, Ray. *Melatonin: Nature's Sleeping Pill*. Be Happier Press, 1995.

Scheffer, Mechthild. *Bach Flower Therapy: Theory and Practice*, Healing Arts Press, 1988.

Segal, Maybelle. *Reflexology*, Wilshire Book Co., 1976.

Sweigard, Lulu E., *Human Movement Potential: Its Ideokinetic Facilitation*, University Press of America, 1988; Harper & Row, 1974.

Teeguarden, Iona M. *Acupressure Way of Health: Jin Shin Do*, Japan Publications, 1978.

About the Author

Janet Diamond has been a New York State licensed massage therapist since 1984. She has a private practice in New York City, as well as working out of such four-star hotels as the Plaza and the Millennium Hilton. She also studies and performs oriental dance. Her full-length plays, one-acts, and comedy sketches have been performed off-off-Broadway and at various cabarets throughout the New York area. She is a resident of New York City.